Six Healing Sounds with Lisa and Ted

For my sister Deirdre

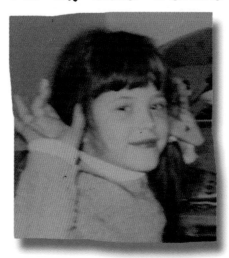

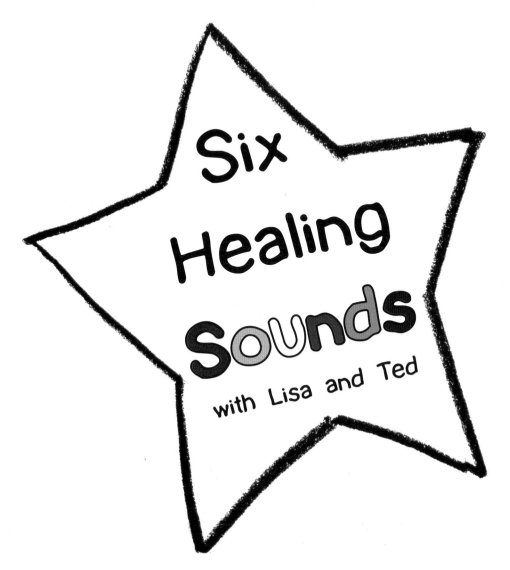

Six

Healing

Sounds

with Lisa and Ted

Qigong for Children

Written and Illustrated by Lisa Spillane

LONDON AND PHILADELPHIA

First published in 2011
by Singing Dragon
an imprint of Jessica Kingsley Publishers

116 Pentonville Road
London N1 9JB, UK
and
400 Market Street, Suite 400
Philadelphia, PA 19106, USA

www.singing-dragon.com

Library of Congress Cataloging-in-Publication Data
Spillane, Lisa.
Six healing sounds with Lisa and Ted : qigong for children / Lisa Spillane.
p. cm.
ISBN 978-1-84819-051-1 (alk. paper)
1. Qi gong--Juvenile literature. I. Title.
RA781.8.S65 2011
613.7'1489--dc22
2010046156

British Library Cataloguing in Publication Data
A CIP catalogue record for this book is available from the British Library

ISBN 978 1 84819 051 1

Printed and bound in India by Replika Press Pvt. Ltd.

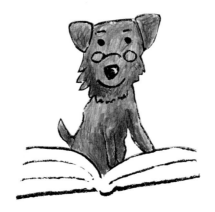

Contents

A Note from the Author

The Six Healing Sounds and Inner Smile exercises were developed thousands of years ago in China to help people to purge toxic negative emotions from their bodies. They've been combined in this book to make a powerful practice that works to heal the body and mind at the same time. The exercises use smiling, deep breathing, vibratory breathing sounds, visualizing and positive thinking with gentle movements, to calm and detoxify the organs. Each organ has its own healing sound, color and set of positive and negative emotions. All of that might sound a bit complicated but Lisa and Ted will show you that it's really very simple.

So why does it work? The practice helps to combat the dangerous effects of stress by activating the body's own healing systems. Put simply, research findings tell us that the exercises work because:

- **breathing deeply** (keeping the shoulders down and allowing the belly area to expand as you inhale and then using the tummy muscles to pull the belly back in as you exhale) calms the body and mind. It also increases the amount of oxygen rich blood which is needed for energy and healing and it boosts the lymphatic system helping it to get rid of toxins

- **smiling** (even when we don't feel like it) strengthens the body's immune system and prompts it to produce hormones that make us feel happy

- **the healing sounds** made while exhaling have a calming, cooling and detoxifying effect on the body's organs

- **thoughts of gratefulness and appreciation** calm the nervous system and protect the heart.

At the core of this practice is a belief that directing loving kindness towards ourselves and others brings healing and emotional tolerance. Lisa and Ted show children that it's natural to have all kinds of emotions and that they can overcome bad feelings by how they think and act. The stories show that being cruel, anxious, self-pitying or jealous makes us feel unwell but choosing to be compassionate, hopeful, brave, appreciative and generous helps us to feel good. The aim of these exercises is not to rid the body of all negative feelings because a certain amount of them are needed. Holding on to feelings of cruelty, worry, despair or jealousy is never healthy but we know that some fear or anger can be beneficial. When faced with emotional upsets, Lisa and Ted consult their "calmer minds" and choose to use the exercises and positive attitudes to make themselves feel better, but that doesn't mean that all of their uncomfortable feelings go away entirely. We see that they have to be determined to do things that may require an act of selflessness or courage before they feel satisfied again. Understanding that feelings come and go and learning ways to cope with the negative ones leads to greater emotional tolerance. Over time these exercises can help children to be more optimistic and open to new experiences through building confidence in their coping skills.

The calming effect of these exercises makes them an excellent preparation for sleep but they can also be done at any time of the day, except directly after eating when only the stomach sound is advisable. It's best to do all the organs (making the sounds at least 3 times) but you can concentrate on just one or as many as you like as long as you remember to do them in the right order. And, if you'd rather not draw attention to yourself, you can make the sound as soft as a whisper and it will still be effective.

Helping children to live more harmoniously by being better connected to themselves, to others and to the beauty of the world they live in is what this book is all about. I hope it brings you and those you share it with peace, joy and good health.

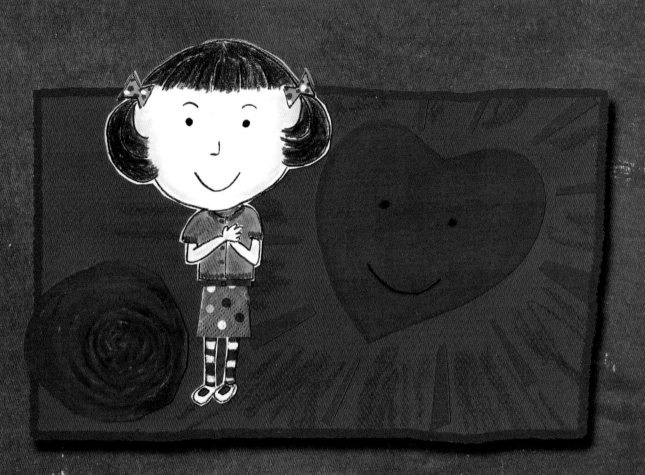

Lisa's Happy Heart

Lisa likes having a happy heart. It fills up with joy when she smiles. Rubbing it warm she says "Thank you heart for pumping blood all around my body." She imagines her heart is red like a beautiful rose and that it's smiling and radiating love as it beats inside her.

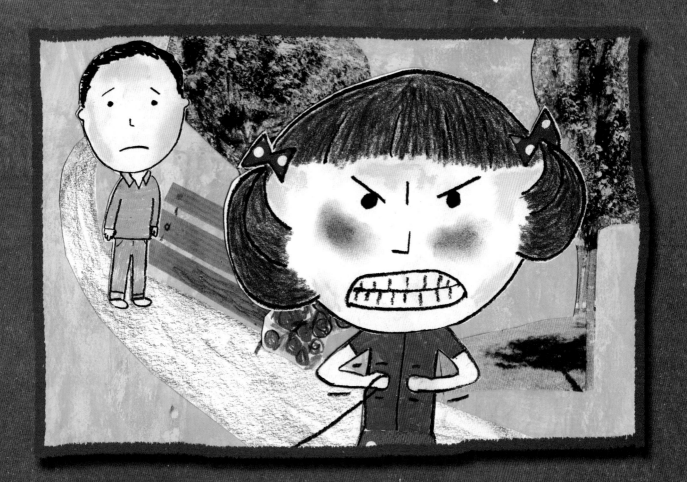

Later on though, Lisa's heart starts to beat faster and harder because she's annoyed at her brother Ted for walking too slow. "Hurry up Ted!" she says angrily. Lisa thinks "When I'm running in a race my heart beats fast and it feels good but when I'm mean to Ted and my heart goes 'bumpety bump...bumpety bump' I feel bad."

She decides to make herself feel better by being patient with Ted. Smiling and taking a deep breath through her nose she breathes in love

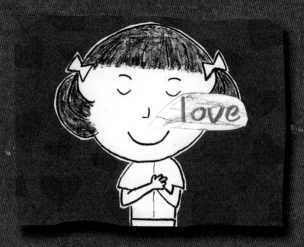

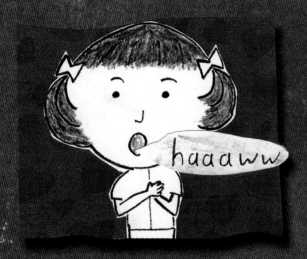

and then breathes out all her impatience and meanness with a **"haaaww"** sound.

With her hand on her heart, she smiles and imagines it full of happiness and love, glowing red like a summer strawberry.

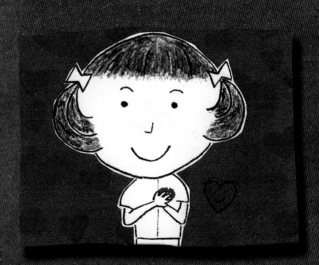

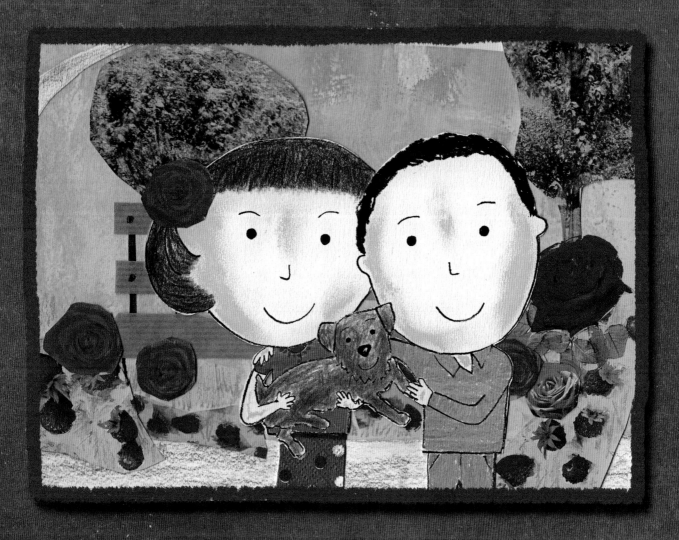

Lisa says "I'm sorry for shouting at you Ted. We
can stop for a rest if you'd like to." Ted gives
her a big smile and Bingo wags his tail.

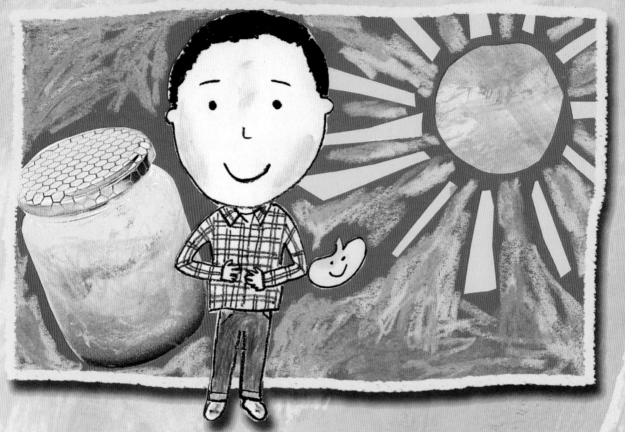

Ted's Friendly Stomach

Ted likes having a friendly stomach. When he smiles it feels really good. Rubbing it warm he says "Thank you stomach for mushing up all the food I eat." He imagines it smiling and glowing with a warm yellow light, like a pot of honey with the sun shining on it.

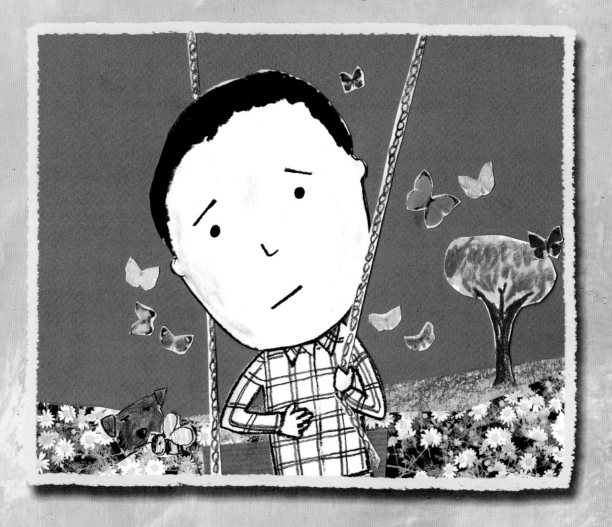

Later on though, Ted's stomach feels upset because he's worried about going to a new school the next day. When he thinks about tomorrow his stomach feels a bit like it does when he's on a swing. He likes being pushed on a swing but he doesn't like feeling worried.

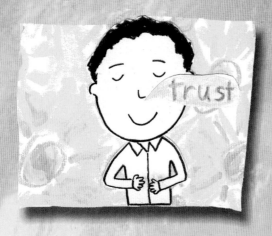

Ted decides not to worry any more. Instead he thinks about how nice it will be to make new friends. He says "I'm going to blow all my worries out of my stomach." Smiling and taking a deep breath through his nose, he breathes in trust

and then breathes out all his worries with a **"whooooooo"** sound.

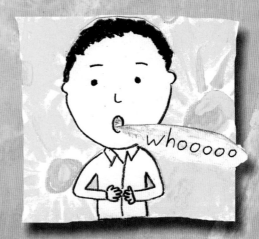

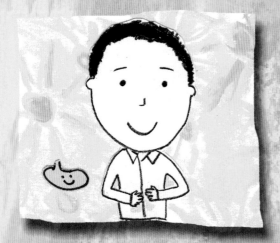

Rubbing his stomach and smiling, Ted imagines it filling up with golden sunlight and he thinks about how good it feels to be friendly.

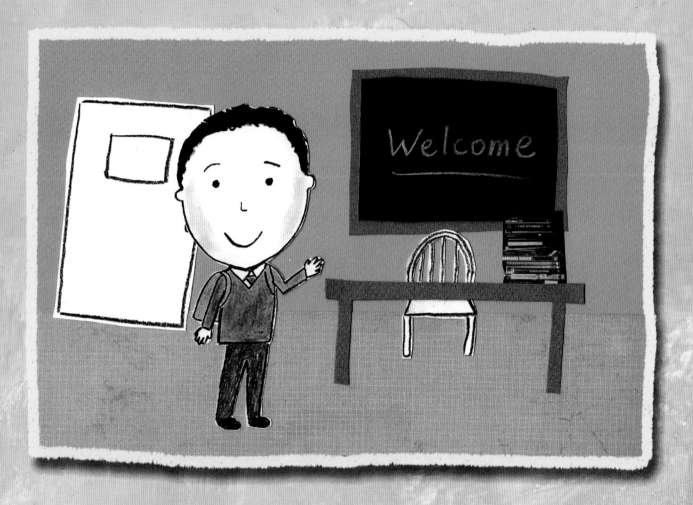

The next day Ted smiles a lot because he has fun meeting all the boys and girls in his class.

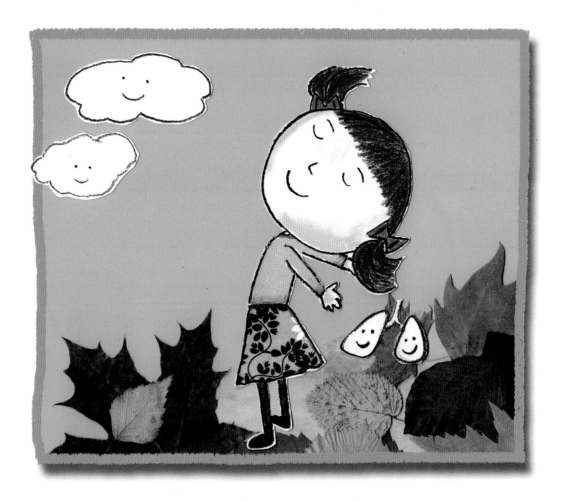

Lisa's Brave Lungs

Lisa likes having brave lungs. They feel full of energy when she smiles. Breathing in fresh air she says "Thank you lungs for bringing air into my body." She imagines her lungs are like two smiling white clouds.

Later on though, Lisa starts to feel sad because she's lonely. Ted is at his friend's house and she has no one to play with. Being sad makes her feel tired. She likes being tired at bedtime but not during the day.

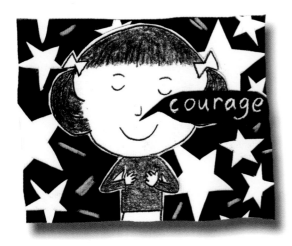

Lisa thinks "I'm going to cheer up." Smiling and taking a deep breath through her nose, she breathes in courage

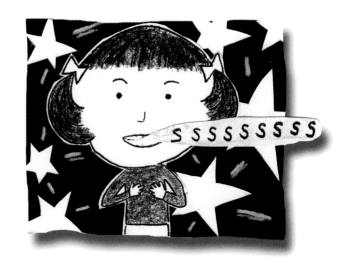

and then breathes out all her sad feelings with a **"SSSSSSSSSSSS"**

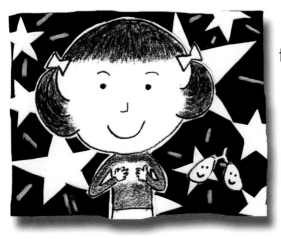

Imagining that she's breathing in twinkling white stars full of courage and thankfulness makes her smile. Feeling the warmth of her hands on her lungs, she thinks about how much fun she has with Ted and about all the people who love her.

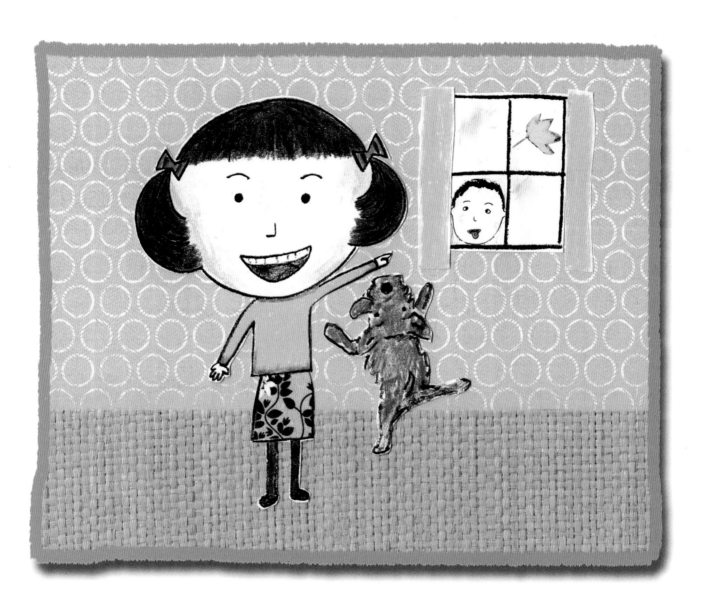

"Ha, ha, ha" laughs Lisa when she sees Ted
making a silly face at the window.

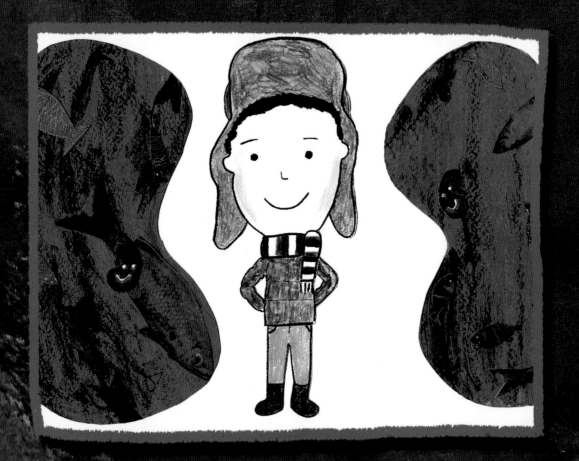

Ted's Peaceful Kidneys

Ted likes having peaceful kidneys. They feel calm when he smiles. Rubbing them warm he says "Thank you kidneys for cleaning my blood." He imagines them smiling and filled with peaceful blue water.

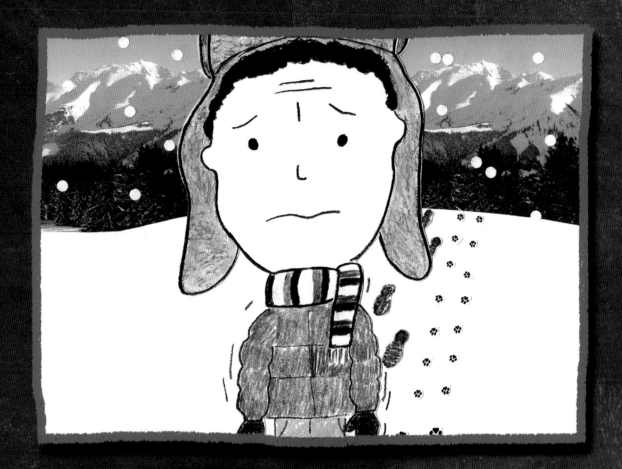

Later on though, he starts to tremble a little because he's afraid of falling off his sleigh. "I *really* want to try it but I'm too scared!" he shouts down the slope to Lisa. Ted knows that it's good to feel frightened sometimes because that feeling warns him to be careful. Now though, he wants to calm down a bit so he can concentrate on getting down the hill.

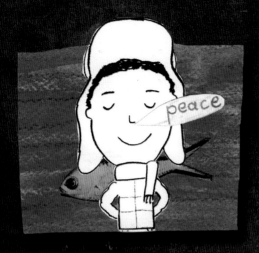

Ted thinks "I can do this because I've sleighed down hills like this before and even if I fall off, the snow is so soft it won't hurt me." Smiling and taking a deep breath through his nose he breathes in peace

and then breathes out his fear with a **"tchewwww"** sound. The small of his back (where his kidneys are) feels cold, so he rubs it warm.

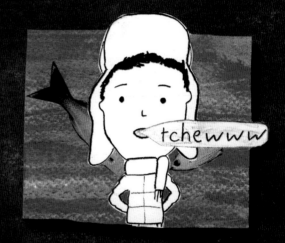

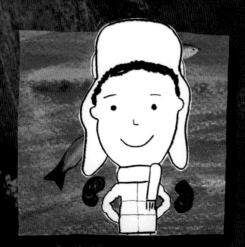

As he smiles, he imagines that his kidneys are like two lakes of calm blue water. Ted still feels a little bit afraid but he's ready to try it.

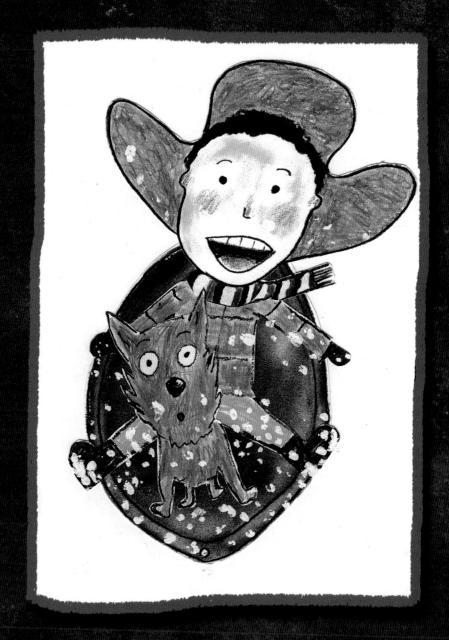

"Ha, ha, ha, he, he, heeeeeeeeee!" Ted laughs
as he sleighs down the hill with Bingo.

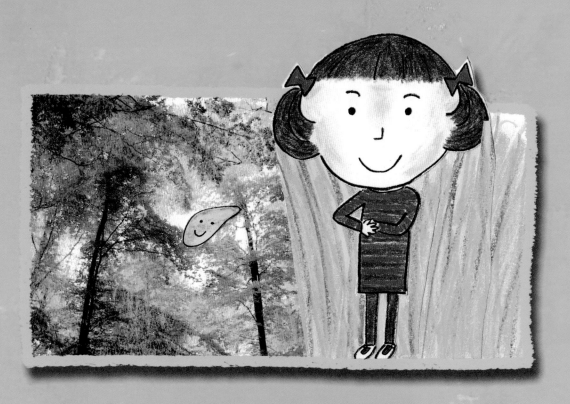

Lisa's Generous Liver

Lisa likes having a generous liver. It feels nice when she smiles and even better when she does something good for someone else. Feeling the warmth of her hand on her liver (which is underneath her ribs on her right side) she says "Thank you liver for making my blood healthy." She imagines it smiling and turning bright green like sunlit grass after the rain.

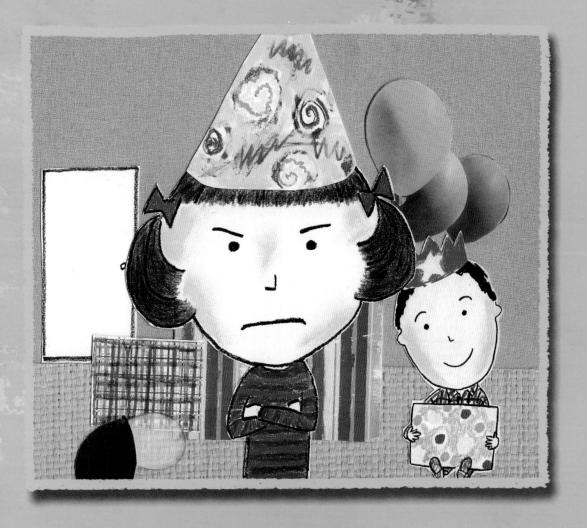

Later on though, Lisa starts to feel grumpy because she's jealous of Ted. It's his birthday and he has lots of presents. She knows that everyone feels jealous sometimes but if she wants to enjoy the party then she will have to try to be happy for Ted.

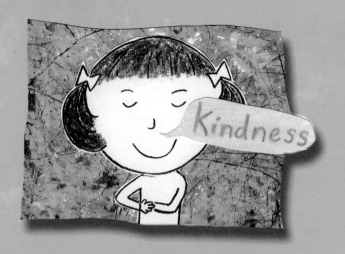

Smiling and taking a deep breath through her nose, she breathes in kindness

and then breathes out all her feelings of jealousy and anger with a **"shhhhh"** sound.

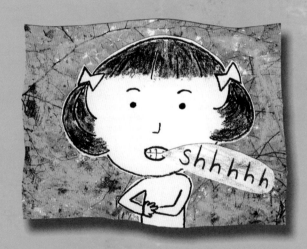

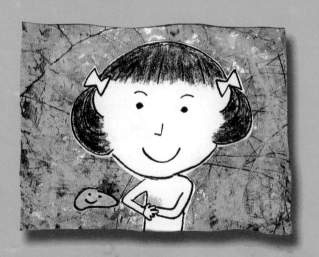

Gently rubbing her liver and smiling, she imagines it filling up with generosity and becoming bright green, like a forest in Spring.

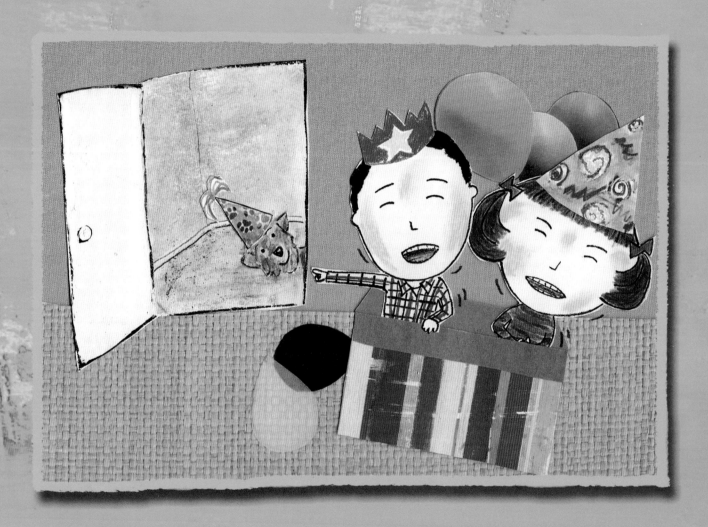

Lisa says "Happy Birthday Ted!" and she gives him his present with a smile. "Ruff, ruff" says Bingo and they both laugh when they see that he's wearing a party hat.

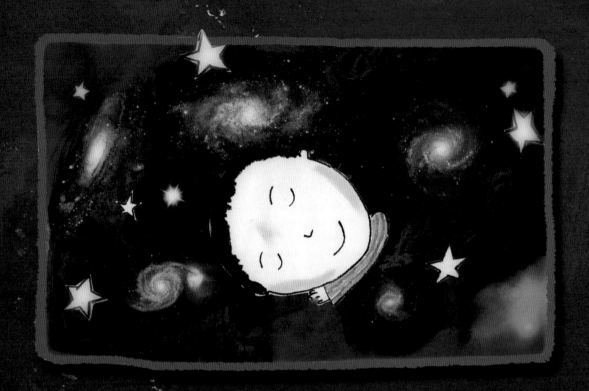

Ted's Sleepy Head

Ted likes having a sleepy head when it's bedtime. His head feels peaceful when he smiles as he drifts off to sleep. Smiling and thinking about good things makes him feel calm and relaxed all over his body. Ted says "Thank you brain for working hard to keep me safe and happy." He imagines his thoughts disappearing in swirling purple light while he snuggles down to sleep.

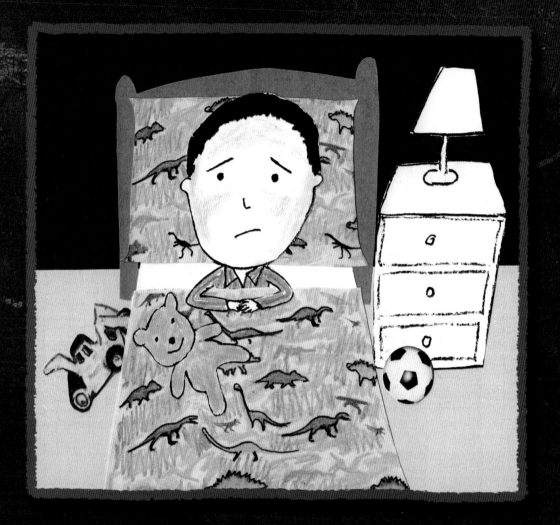

Tonight though, Ted's brain is keeping him awake with busy
thoughts. His head feels hot, his heart is beating quickly
and he's not comfortable in his bed. Ted thinks "I'm glad
that my mind does a lot of thinking during the day but
now I want it to be quiet so I can relax and go to sleep."

Lying on his back with his arms at his side and the palms of his hands facing up, he takes a deep breath through his nose while raising his arms above his head. As he slowly brings his arms back down he breathes out his busy thoughts with a **"heeeeee"** sound.

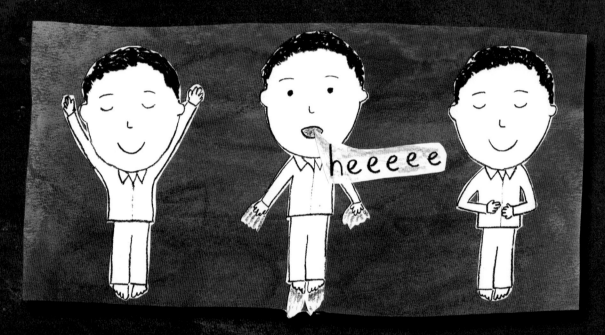

Ted pretends when he's breathing out that his hands are pushing warm purple light down his body. He pictures the chattering noise from his head turning into dark smoke that leaves him through the tips of his fingers and toes. Feeling calm and relaxed, he rests his hands on his stomach.

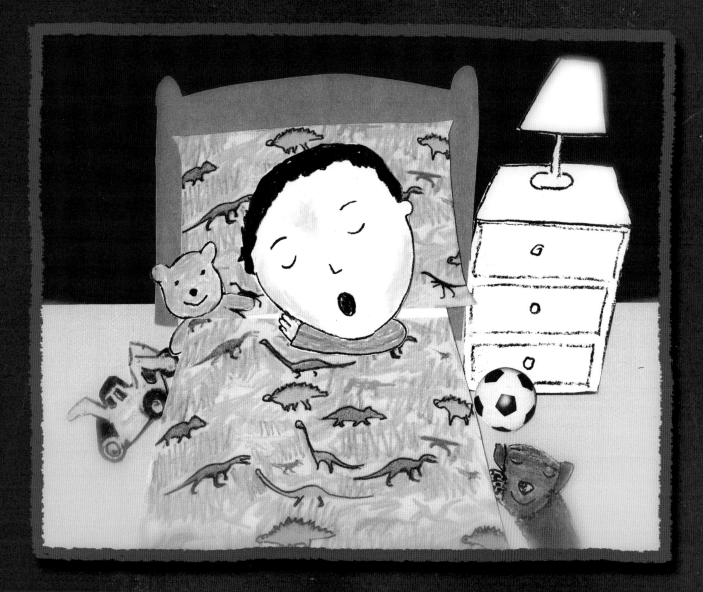

Now Ted's head feels cool and very sleepy. His heart is beating gently and his feet are cosy and warm. After a little yawn he falls fast asleep.

of related interest

The Chinese Book of Animals
Chungliang Al Huang
ISBN 978 1 84819 066 5

Qigong Massage for Your Child with Autism
A Home Program from Chinese Medicine
Louisa Silva
ISBN 978 1 84819 070 2